THE LAST RESORT

A NOVELLA IN VOICES

ALLIE COKER

ISBN: 978-1-7358600-9-1

Coker. Allie.
The Last Resort.

Editing: Melissa Long

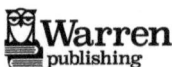

Warren publishing

Published by Warren Publishing
Charlotte, NC
www.warrenpublishing.net
Printed in the United States

For the lost ones, here and gone.
You will find your way.
You will be remembered.

And for Ned, Tara, and Jeff.

AUTHOR'S NOTE

Due to the sensitive subject matter in *The Last Resort*, I've included a list of trigger warnings for readers who may need them:

- discussion of mental health—portrayals of depression, panic attacks, schizophrenia, anxiety
- discussion and description of suicide
- description of physical abuse
- description of self-harm
- description of mental facility

I also wish to recognize that mental health and illness are not a monolithic experience. The opinions, thoughts, and feelings portrayed in this work of fiction are not meant to represent an entire population or community, or account for all individual experiences.

PREFACE

When I chose to accept the offer for my first corporate job, it was a positive change. I had just finished being a full-time caregiver, had separated from my relationship, and had no car, license, or substantial work history. I had to buy professional attire and take a taxi to my interviews. Once I began working, I moved to an apartment complex within walking distance of my job, which made me slightly more independent. The job gave me a purpose, fresh goals, and a built-in support system. It took some stress off my loved ones I'm sure, but it also made those around me notice how important work was to me. It made me notice too.

Business Allie grew up within those walls, learning from the best, discovering distinct work values, and taking note of it all. I got a license, bought a car, and closed on a house—I was a bonafide adult by all the usual demarcations, despite being a late bloomer where acquiring a license and job history were concerned. The job held meaning for me because I could directly track it back to my days as a caregiver for my ailing spouse, dressing wounds and administering IV antibiotics, as well as my own troubled medical history. Having insights to the medical world—either as a patient, caregiver, or advocate since I was five years old—gave me decades of experience when it came to knowing about medications and how quickly they should arrive from home health. In some ways, it felt like I had been preparing for my position my whole life. It was almost enough to distract me from my lifelong passion—writing.

I started my career in May 2014, but my dream of over twenty years was realized in the form of a diploma in June 2014, when I earned my MFA in creative writing. Of course, I had been a writer all along and had even published a book two years prior to graduating, but sometimes self-knowledge takes a (long) moment to catch up to reality. In a country that so staunchly follows a two-part value judgment system—you're either a starving artist or a banker but seldom an entity that overlaps—I began to see the concept of "passion" in a new light. Yes, it was the blurry idea that fueled my waking dreams, but it was also what I felt for my everyday job. It occurred to me that just as we are capable of loving more than one person at a time—our partner, our parents/children, our best friend—we are capable of holding several passions in our heart.

That simple concept embodies all that I've tried to impart in this novella. There are multiple dimensions to a person, a situation, an institution—even if our rigid definitions confine us to believe otherwise. Things are not always what they seem, but the invisible line we all draw in our heads between "us" and "them," "normal" and "defective" is just that—invisible, unnecessary, and unhelpful in our attempts to understand one another and ourselves. This novella is my battle cry, my imploration, my entreaty, and my invitation. My two passions cannot balance or exist without each other, and I am grateful for both.

PART ONE
THE LAST RESORT

What name do we put to an instinct
greater than survival?

#19145: The truth is a muddied thing. To begin with, there's so little of it.

#28439: They don't have magic answers like we thought they would. Lex works her way around her problems but finds no relief. We thought for sure we had just done something wrong, but no one could tell us what. They make us attend AA. One of the guys says that's one good thing about being locked up—it keeps us clean. If I weren't here, I'd be injecting fire into my veins right now, reeling on my back stoop, eyelids fluttering and the neighbors pretending not to notice again. When people can, they walk back and forth, over and over again, trying to make the small courtyard work for them, pacing the concrete and soaking in sunshine, peering through the narrow spaces between wooden slats of the impossibly high fence—perhaps not so impossible since escapees have scaled it before. The courtyard can't be mistaken for a park, not even a garden, but if a stiff breeze blows the right way and you sit close to each other at the picnic table, just shooting the shit, you can imagine a hot July night with friends on the patio and beers in hand. Some people just stand planted in one spot, their arms out, as though they are solar powered.

Napping during the day in your room isn't allowed since you have to be with the group where they can see you. A blanket is dragged every now and then through the halls, wrapped around the shoulders of a person too cold or tired to talk. The hard plastic couch—the same material as a child's playset and initially an object of disgust—turned into the welcoming down of the plushest comforter after a few days. Swaddled and with their backs to us—a true sign of not caring—many sleep for hours until it is time for the group to go to dinner or rec therapy. You see a lot of tired people, napping people, but that is because their bodies are adjusting. It looks very similar to what you would imagine, but that's just it—you have to get past looks.

Lex taught us about the ugly laws and how people used to get separated from society for doing regular stuff like cheating on your girl or being lazy. One moment, you could be reading a book in a hammock and then the next—*bam*! Behind lock and key. She told us about how places like this one were shut down in the '70s. Lex knows a lot of stuff like that. A lot of people say she could work here, could have a key to the locked doors, if only she loved herself more. Lex talks about work a lot. She talks about how fast she can type and how she loves solving problems. She told us about her coworkers and how familial they are. She talks about the difficulty of making sure everything goes just right at her job every single day. For almost every topic, Lex has a work story. I used to wonder what she did to be brought here in handcuffs like the rest of us. I used to think it was a boy, but it turns out it was a lot of people and a lot of circumstances that put her here.

She says her name's Sandy, but I call her Lex. We all call her Lex now. Sandy sounds like a fragile name, wishy-washy, a name that clings to your skin, and I figure if she were that fragile, she'd be a lot meaner. I call her Lex after Lex Luther because he's the whip-smart but evil guy who brought down Superman. Lex isn't evil, but obviously some part of her is filled with hate, mostly for herself. Plus, she talks about work a lot. Like it's her life or something.

Every day, we wait to see who will get out next. They escort us back to our hall, and as the door swings open, I yell, "Cellblock Four West!" Lex hushes me when I do that. She hushes me a lot. She's talkative here, but I think she has trouble sleeping. Whenever she falls asleep in the rec room, she tosses and turns, her jaw set tight as her mind grinds away.

A steel toilet with no lid or seat, a flimsy toothbrush, and thirty seconds of shower water at a time—that's all you get. Waking up to that cold, metal rim and having to ask someone to unlock the shower door for you is its own wake-up call. Shampoo is rare, and razors are out of the question, so prepare to get furry. The only way you get a razor is if someone watches you while you shave, which is too creepy to even think about. Doors lock behind you for every ten feet or so of hallway to prevent drift, lag, and loss. Every piece of furniture is made of bulky plastic—unlikely to be thrown. When group and art therapy happen, we're not allowed to have real pencils, just the stubby kind you get at a minigolf course. Why they think a small pencil would hurt any less when stabbed in your eye, I have no clue. Pens aren't allowed either.

One kid yells. All he does is yell and talk to no one in particular. *All. The. Time.* There's something really wrong with that kid. I say "kid," but we're all adults here, at least in the eyes of the law. When they take our vitals every day, I always try to beat the young ones by getting the lowest blood pressure. Nothing like a little friendly competition to help make light of our situation, I guess.

Some of them are only in their twenties or younger! How'd they end up here so fast? What did life do to them so quickly? I'm triple their age and would never think of doing that stuff. My blood pressure runs kinda high, but I still do my best—sit still, stay calm. H.D. had to break up a bad fight the other day—some kid swinging and attacking anybody near him. They threw him in solitary. The lights go on and off, but there's no doorknob inside, even though we can watch him through the window. Some people are just outta their minds. Sure, I wanted to hurt people, but that was different. They were chasing me.

H.D.: I try my best to help them. After all, I could just as easily end up here one day. My night shift relief, Cameron, makes the rounds every fifteen minutes, which includes checking who's asleep and marking their position to make sure they're not trying to harm themselves or those in the room with them. I stay up and review like a worried camp counselor. Who spoke in group today? Who responded to rec time or pet therapy?

Who isn't eating? Who is beating their head on the wall again? It's surprising to me to see so many oldsters in here. They're easily two to three decades older than me, and I'm not a spring chicken—more of a middle-aged rooster.

Sometimes the system makes me feel useless. Sure, there are others in my position who don't care. They look and sound bored and do the bare minimum of watching the group to ensure they don't escape. But if you're not here to help people, then why do it? This job may not be glamorous or joyful, but sometimes I think the world is twice as messed up on the outside. I truly believe I could easily end up on this unit one day, taking timed showers with push buttons, not being able to see the outside world without a fence, eating the same meals on rotation with plastic silverware. There's nothing special about any of us that prevents us from slipping; we're all susceptible. I just try to do a little bit of good, to help them some. You can always tell who will end up back here though. This batch seems like a cakewalk compared to some. One guy we had in last month—well, we'll see him again.

#80912: I do *not* belong here. They should have just sent me back home to handle my problems on my own— that's the reasonable thing to do. Here, everyone looks at me funny. They think I don't notice, but I do.

The first three days of my stay, I walked past the locked door with trepidation. Some kind of confinement room meant for a single occupant. A cell where the lights and locks are controlled from the *outside*—somehow used to calm people down (supposedly). There was a creepy little window that bowed in and seemed out of place on the door. The light stayed off, and the door stayed locked. Some of the long-term residents—imagine being here for more than a month!—told me that's where Boris stays, describing him as a hulking, six-foot-five guy with shoulders that barely fit through the doorway and tattoos on his eyelids. His silence is so thick you could choke on it. Lured in, I kept trying to peek until my third day. My heart thumped rapidly the closer I edged to the door with the darkened, concave window. Finally, I got so close that the toes of my shoes almost lined up with the doorframe. Almost. One of those girl loonies with long, blond hair came up behind me, lightly tapped my shoulders, and yelled, "Boo!" My eardrum exploded, and an electric pulse jutted through my neck and into my skull. My heart drummed triple time. That's when I knew Boris wasn't real at all. Should have known better than to listen to a bunch of nuts.

They're almost as bad as the nurses who all whisper about me at night. They think I don't know, but I can hear them. They're trying to keep me here when I don't need to be here. I hear snatches of their hushed conversations. They won't use my name, but when they say "she" and "her," I know they mean me. I need to get back to my life, which has been falling apart rapidly. My significant other of three years started cheating on me six months ago, though he'll never admit it. He's working more hours than before, and once a week, he leaves the house with his buddies to go "bowling." When he comes back a few hours later, smiling and cheerful as he gloats over the scorecard he shows me, I wonder how much he had to pay some dumb schmuck to obtain it. Two of my coworkers have been making me look bad to the boss and are trying to push me out. They deny everything. That's what I don't get about people—why do they deny so much?

G.K.: People I meet outside my job always assume the patients I work with claim they're George Washington or an alien from deep space. Or they think I work with kids who levitate and speak in forty-three different tongues—they've seen all the movies. While there certainly are people who may fit those descriptions and need critical help, the people I tend to work with are usually disturbed in a different way. They are people who can function in society until one day they can't.

H.D. and I talk about what it means to be a mental health worker a lot. Where the line between responsibility and administering techniques, guidance, and solution-oriented thinking blurs. It's different from being a therapist or a nurse, though there's certainly overlap at times. Our job is to aid them in developing coping skills—along with the help of therapy and meds—so they can return to society and never be committed again, if possible. If they return, we will greet them warmly and help them once more, knowing their relapse is not a personal failing but rather a nasty trick of biology.

T.J.: One thing that surprised me when I first started working here was the amount of laughter people find in such a dismal situation. Granted, if they can laugh, they shouldn't be here, in my opinion. It's all in their heads anyway. H.D. and G.K. play the saintly roles, but I feel more like security personnel than anything else. These people have been stripped of their rights for a reason! But many have formed a code or secret bond. You see them making bizarre hand gestures at each other while I hand out worksheets or hear them whispering conspiratorially while I begin giving instructions for our breathing exercises. Right, 'cause breathing is really gonna help this pack of fools! Razzing the new kid brings them a certain amount of joy—or else the new kid comes out swinging, to which their response is to leave them alone.

They had one new recruit—if this were the draft, that is—tiptoeing around the quiet room for days, spinning some tale about Boris, who never really existed. They howled about it for days and at the most inopportune times, collapsing on their backsides during yoga or busting a gut after cutting each other sidelong glances during group. "Hey," one of them would call during a downward dog, their compatriot across the room looking up just long enough from their sweaty mat to catch the mouthed word "Bo-ris" with overexaggerated syllables and a smile brighter than the 40-watt bulbs used in this facility. Giggles erupt. I am in a room full of adults who are enjoying themselves immensely. No one told them to stop though—not the yoga instructors or rec technician. Certainly not me. There's too much pain in this world to forbid laughter, and if these idiots want to yuck it up, who am I to stop them?

G.K.: When you're a kid and life should be light, grown-ups and teachers all want you to be serious. "Pipe down!" they say. They squelch the laughter. But ironically, what's acceptable when you're a kid becomes an absolute curse on the lips of others as you age—whether true or not. You like rainbow colors? Gay. You have an imaginary friend? Insane. You love making crafts? Starving artist. We take something so innocent and beautiful and ruin it. I'm surprised we all don't end up here as a refuge from the harsh world at some point or another. Let them laugh about Boris all they want. So many things start out beautiful and turn ugly, it's almost nice to have the opposite be true for once. They talk a lot about Lex, too, but I've never met someone here named that.

H.D.: A lot of my friends ask me how I can stand to be around crazy people all day. In return, I ask them how they can stand to be around me. They laugh, but I always follow it up with, "Seriously." They see my eyebrows arched high and know I'm not joking.

I climb up on my soapbox, a practiced and measured hop that still takes all the energy I have. I tell them that people who *choose* to be in the lives of those with mental illness share a common denominator of some sort. Sure, it takes patience, emotional fortitude, and, at times, an unrealistic amount of compassion, but I know that as someone in a good mental state, I'm no cakewalk to be around either. People are people, sick or not. I remind friends that defining someone solely by their diagnosis is as shortsighted as constantly referring to others as Green-eyed Mary or Surfer Mark. Aren't we more than just the sum of our parts? Surely we should be just as interested in the occupation, family life, hobbies, and beliefs of a cancer patient as we are in the fact that they have cancer. Just like cancer, mental illness is not a choice. Sure, we do things that help or harm our mental state every day, but in the end, the verdict is handed down by nerves and neurons, not some deficiency in spirit or willpower.

My friends, having gotten way more than what they've asked for, wait silently, unsure of how to react. "So who's really crazy?" I ask. "Because I do *choose* to live with something I don't even have." During my training, I did some research on "depressive realism." It's the belief that those who are depressed actually see the world more accurately than the rest of us. I don't know if that's true or not, but I do know that there are more than two ways to look at things.

They look like they want to kick the soapbox out from under me. Instead, I hop down, quickly, by myself.

T.J.: I don't know why some of the others take this so seriously. These people are just a bunch of assholes who got themselves into this mess anyway. Give me a break. This isn't an illness; it's a choice. My aunt Viola is dying of neck cancer back on Long Island. *That's* an illness.

#66921: I like being here better than being at home. At home, there was never anything to do or anywhere to go. I guess because it wasn't my home in the first place. At least here, I get three square meals a day and no one's constantly beating me. The people who made us this way should be in here. They push you to the edge and then you break, and they get to walk away freely. No one makes them seek help. It just ain't right.

G.K.: Routine seems to be a big deal for those recovering or coping with physical and mental changes. This is reinforced when you see schedules in physical rehabilitation centers, senior citizen homes, and mental hospitals—prisons too.

#28439: Her eyes flash darkly sometimes, and I can tell if it's going to be a Superman moment or a Lex moment. People think kryptonite is Superman's only weakness, and Lex is just a nemesis. What they don't realize is that Lex can be both. I'm pretty sure Sandy can feel it—the dark path of her mind, the looping spirals that lead her further and further down until her body feels as heavy as her soul. She can feel the shimmer of it coming on, but she only gets angry if she tries to push past it, repel it—it's a weakness she must bow to time and time again. Her mind is her own worst enemy. I can hear the shift in her normally cheerful voice to a tone that's tinged with impatience before she gets to a point of sheer anger. She doesn't take it out on us so much as she seems fed up with her charade that everything's fine when, clearly, it isn't. It's not unlike a child's tantrum at times.

#91185: She acts very serious, like she's apart from the rest of us in some way. When she talks, though, I doubt she's ever truly seen a hard day in her life. Then again, she could be hiding things. Sometimes, she talks about her brother, but a few of us heard she's an only child.

#66921: It was the worst idea of my life. The hardwood was clammy underneath my perspiring body. The day had been too long. Halfway through my turkey with cranberry sauce and my cousin's long-winded explanation of how and why he was so successful, I excused myself upstairs to the bathroom and didn't come back.

I stared into the mirror for two and a half minutes; anyone I had ever loved was downstairs, and yet I knew they wouldn't find me until the evening, after the dishes had been unceremoniously stacked in the sink, the leftovers gnawed on, and the postgame debrief ended. They would assume I was napping or having one of my anxiety spells but would not actually bother to check. I'm a wimp about pain, and my orange, plastic razor has a guard, so the lines I made were thin and jagged but deep. Drops of crimson dotted the floor beside my bed as I lay down—no longer any need for comfort. I stared at the popcorn ceiling and dark varnish of my bureau. *Just slip away.* I got up with considerable effort and ran my wrists under warm water, pinching the sides to extract more blood—the raw slashes already looked angry. I didn't feel great.

As I lay back down, the blood pooling more effectively now, my last thoughts were around the raises I didn't get, the lengthy stints of unemployment and job hopping I had to go through, and the fact that I would not be showing up on Monday to my temp assignment that I, by some miracle, passed the drug test to obtain. For ten years since I'd left college, I'd been on the straight and narrow. My position at the firm demanded that of me, filled me with purpose and more than one reason to stay alert. The day I was fired came as a complete shock. "Downsizing," they said. "You understand how hard it is in this economy."

You understand how hard it is in this economy. I didn't then as the words rang in my ears, but being let go taught me just how hard the economy was out there. A security guard walked me to my desk at the end of the day. "You're a good employee. It's just procedure," the firm manager informed me.

It's just procedure. I sobbed into my steering wheel as I drove to my cousin's house, the only relative who had enough space to put me up for a while. I drove myself to what would become a cage of fear and rage—my fear and his rage at having to put up with a good-for-nothing relative. Each dish washed improperly, each shirt with a wrinkle, each weed that escaped me turned into a physical battle where he, inevitably, came out the victor. Since then, I had revisited my green friend many times. It was the only thing that kept the panic at bay. Plus, it's not like it's a real drug, so no problem. Life sober was unnecessary and unfruitful. My last fading thought was that I was an ugly person, eclipsed by the faint sound of my aunt politely knocking on the door.

#**91185** I think about death more than the average person. Heck, as a hospice nurse, I'm confronted with it every day. I did fine until Dad was dying. All the platitudes in the world won't bring him back. Simpler to leave before he does. I was gripped by an indifference to life so strong it choked me. I have a hard time trusting myself, let alone others.

#28439: Fifty years together, and I was being left. I wasn't as good as the damn cat. I pondered my shotgun, jumping, and simply laying down and dying, but none of it struck a chord. What did was hearing the crisp edict of, "I'm locking the door and taking Cuppy. I've left your *stuff*." Click.

Lights out, curtain down on the one relationship that defined my whole life. It wasn't like there was a falling out. Had I been unkind? Vicious? Unfair? Probably, at times—more than I needed to be at least. But to not even be given a reason or a warning—well, that was too damn much. I exploded. Hearing the stiff message on my mobile phone was the last straw.

I've left your stuff.

I've left your stuff.

I've left your stuff.

My foot pressed down harder and harder with each iteration. I rounded the country curve, the stop sign flying past me, the empty road ahead. Sixty-six. Seventy-five. Ninety.

I'm locking the door.

I veered right and aimed for an ancient pine. And then I woke up in a room that was not my own.

#00639: My twin followed me everywhere like a shadow. Even though I was not the favorite, even though I was never cool, everywhere I went, there were two of me. I started drinking for two in high school, my church at the time pushing harder and harder for us to get confirmed. I knew I was trapped because I held the salvation of two people in my hand and not just one. If I didn't do it, my twin would go to hell. If I did, I'd be a liar and still go to hell.

Just because my twin copied me did not mean we were of the same mind, and when it came to religion—any at all—there was no talking my way out of it, no matter how ardently I lacked belief. I longed for a way out when I cried in bed most nights under the weight of it. I imagined myself on fire—what hell would feel like when I got there. I imagined myself suffocating, pretending to gasp and choke as I envisioned myself trying to denounce it all in front of my parents. I wretched for no reason and was a wretch for no reason. I started taking crazy risks, like walking barefoot across construction zones. Then, when my twin begged me to finally decide "Hadn't we waited long enough? All our other friends were baptized and confirmed long ago!" and pled for me to save our souls, I was twenty-two and couldn't take it anymore.

I knew the exact face I was looking for—big, sloppy muzzle long, droopy ears. The shelter kept such animals contained—and only momentarily—under lock and key in the back. I sidestepped the smell of ammonia as I punched in my volunteer code and made my way back to the rattling cage, but it wasn't rattling. The beast was asleep. At least, I hoped the deed hadn't been done yet. I needed its help. In an uncharacteristic act, one that shocked even me, I delivered a swift kick to the cage, waking the dog within it. I wiggled my fingers between the bars, baiting him. I wasn't interested in repeat performances. I wasn't interested in anything anymore.

My twin screamed at me, started pacing angrily and yelling the passionate cry of someone who is both upset and concerned, like a parent finding a lost child who has wondered off. I had just told them the truth, given them the good news. They would be able to get confirmed and join in God's ranks one day ... without me. I didn't have to worry anymore about pulling them down with me because I wouldn't be around to muck things up. By refusing treatment, I had sealed my fate to a cool month at most. It was my decision though, my choice to make it a death sentence. My twin stopped pacing and stared at me, the tears of rage spilling over in her eyes. "But listen—" was all I got out before hearing the stairs creak under my twin's tennis shoes and my own flesh and blood announcing to our parents that I was going to die.

#63630: I only agreed to come because they threatened to take away my cell phone. Big liars. They took it away inside the hospital anyway! I didn't see what all the fuss was about. I was losing weight; I was looking good. They told me to pack two relaxed outfits—I rolled my eyes—and none of my deodorant, shampoo, mouthwash, makeup, or hairspray. Please, like I was going to *eat* deodorant.

"You need to speak to the nurse," my history professor told me during office hours. "There's obviously something going on, and I know this is uncomfortable for us both, but I need you to go."

Big fucking meddler. He would have kept badgering me otherwise, so I went. I had lost fifty pounds in nine weeks. I was working out for two hours each day and only joining my friends for lunch—a PB&J, one of the richest, fattiest, carb-loaded, and sugar-filled meals I could throw together and take to the quad with me for an hour.

"You're so pretty! I wish I could look like you," Antonia chirped.

"Oh no," I'd demure. "I eat awful," I'd say, pointing to the enemy sandwich. I hated that I had to eat it at all, but I got shaky and weak while jogging if I didn't. So what if my clothes had gotten a little baggy? I looked good and felt fine—just wasn't hungry. Besides, I obviously had plenty more to lose. What did they know? That fucking professor wouldn't have noticed me at all—or at least would have noticed me like he noticed Michelle—if I were thinner and prettier ....

#19145: I have known love, and I have known fear. To me, they feel the same.

#80912'S FILE, RELATIVE REPORT: I could see the round, white, cylindrical cap pried off and lying limp on the leather seat. The sun blazed through the orange bottle, spilling irradiated sunlight down to the floorboard. I banged on the window—harder than I meant to. It made an unsatisfying, hollow sound as I smacked it. Then I kept banging and crying out. Finally, after fumbling it once onto the concrete, I used my phone to dial 911. The only number where someone answers on the first ring. The only number that never changes. The glossed-over eyes combined with the overwhelming heat inside the car pushed my sense of urgency as I pressed my palm hard against the glass.

OFF US-19, WEST VIRGINIA: He was so high he couldn't remember his own name. Charlie? Chandler? He knew he was a DeWitt, but which one? His feet sidled up to the edge of the bridge, and he noted how they seemed to move independent of one another. Below him, far below him, the midnight blue waves curdled and swirled, rushing freely with the autumn wind. For a split second, scenes from Jimmy Stewart's most famous film flashed in his mind. It wasn't too late; he could still go home. Friends he didn't know he had, friends from nowhere, would turn out, a small fortune would turn up, Zuzu would feel better, and the sun would always shine. He leapt, and while he wouldn't make it off this mortal coil, he would be paralyzed from the waist down for the rest of his sorry life.

H.D.: My job keeps me up a lot at night. My fiancée usually rolls over to a sunken blanket somewhere between 2:15 and 2:48 a.m. to find me gone, her rusty voice softly calling my name in the dark. Like generations before me, I sit at the kitchen table worrying—not about bills or the kids we don't have but about complete strangers.

I'm not naïve. I know two, three, four weeks can't fix their lives, that their improvements while in the institution may or may not hold up under pressure once they are released. I'd like to do more, but I'm just one person, and I'm not even sure where to start. How do you teach someone the bare necessities of survival once they're past the first two decades? That's not to say we don't make a difference—the rate of harm to oneself or others would be much higher without our social/clinical services. It's just difficult to know whether you've gotten through to someone or not. Like working with cancer patients, it's emotionally scarring to hear someone has left your facility and passed. Of course, most of the time we don't hear anything unless we're laying eyes on them in person again.

My first was Jay. He was a good kid, deep thinker, a parent's dream except for the cuts up and down his inner arm, a way to punish himself for being "bad"—a slipped grade, a bully parroting a remark back to him, a passing doubt about the order of this universe. He took his meds without complaint, participated heavily in all the groups, and even befriended some of the other patients, always trying to include them. He smiled and deemed himself more or less cured the last day of his two weeks here, and then he walked off and killed himself. I guess we can never really know someone, not truly. According to the kitchen table at two in the morning, I barely even know myself. We got a thank you letter from Jay's parents. This is rare. Usually we're accused of not fixing someone's son or daughter, spouse or sibling. The issue is that these people are just like everyone else—they don't need fixing—just extra help, gentle guidance, to get back to living their best lives as their best selves. God, I'm starting to sound like a self-help book. Maybe I should just quit.

DEPUTY JOHNS: If you think it gets boring, repetitive, and lonesome, well, you'd be right. The same empty seat to my right, tons of cornfields to my left—for hours, for three hundred miles. Four days a week, fifty weeks a year. The radio signal is strong on my Charger, and for that, I'm grateful because small talk is out of the question most times. It's an odd job, shepherding people to places they don't want to go. Less of a taxi situation and more like a benevolent kidnapper. They have to trust me even though, by all measures, I convey I don't trust them. Hence the handcuffs. Hence the shield. Hence the fact that I have to sign for the person at the origination and destination sites as though I just got a package from UPS.

G.K.: I'm not so sure the program works. Is reading the Bible going to make someone else stop beating you? Is petting a dog going to stop your cravings for amphetamines? Sure, you can't smoke in here, but what are we teaching to help the cessation postrelease? I guess the idea is to give the mind a respite. Stop it from spinning in the same cycle nonstop eight plus hours a day. Distraction can be a wonderful technique when used properly and with a healthy habit. Chewing gum, not binge eating. Taking up a sport instead of allowing your anger issues to ruin you. Things like that. But the whole promise of things getting better is a coin toss. The trick is, things may get worse, but how equipped will these people be to handle them? That's the only modicum of control we have in this life.

#91185: It wasn't snowing. Sixty-five degrees and sunny on Christmas Day—it could have been California except landlocked. The surrounding houses' buzz of excitement had quieted as their smallest inhabitants poured over their newfound bounty early in the morning.

8:45 a.m. I thought of Brinker, but it was too early to call. Pajamas still on, I padded downstairs to make a strong cup of coffee and some egg whites. I glanced at a book as I ate my eggs and quietly decided what to do next.

9:15 a.m. The mall opened at 10:00 a.m. but was a good forty minutes away. I wiped my mouth and plugged in the tree. It lit up bleakly, straining under the shadow of not enough lights—another strand or two would have done—but it was no matter now. Barren underneath, the tree was barely a presence. Two unopened envelopes lay on my coffee table. I ripped through the cranberry red envelope of the first to uncover a form letter, the smiling faces of two toddlers beaming up at me. "Love, the Allisters." The second was a short note from Vance. "Hope your holidays are wonderful!"

My lips turned up slightly. I refilled my coffee mug and peered through the blinds—no one in sight but a wreath adorning every door. Marching back upstairs to brush my teeth, I missed a step and set my heart to racing. "Damn," I whispered. The cat slid by me, its body a furry locomotive gaining momentum the closer it got to the landing. After buttoning my pants and pulling on the one Christmas sweater I owned, I fished my keys out from the drawer.

10:05 a.m. It was hard to believe the mall was open on Christmas Day, but there it was, commerce at its best. Even the Chik-Fil-A was open, which I found odd given their Sunday practices. I took a loop around the desolate mall before parking myself at a table in the food court. Empty on any given day, this mall had been struggling for years. I wasn't the only one there though. A family of six packed in around the table in front of mine, all of them in equally garish sweaters. And of course, there were the mall employees. I couldn't raise my spirits enough to cash in on all the holiday deals happening around me, so after a couple hours of sauntering around aimlessly, I made the forty-minute trek home.

1:15 p.m. I called Brinker and left a voicemail, then I sent a few texts to a couple other people. There was a three o'clock showing of a sci-fi movie I'd wanted to see, so I took a short nap before leaving the house again. It could have been any other unremarkable day—not the birth of a savior, the final holiday of the year, or a day for kith and kin. It could have been the Tuesday after a bad Saturday-night hangover. The movie was decent but centered around a love story more than I thought it should. When I got back, it was past five o'clock in the evening, and the dark had settled. No porch light was left on for me.

PART TWO

LEX

LEX: In my county, the jailbirds get phones in every cell, pens to write with, and fresh local eggs. Apparently, the cuckoos do not. We are the wrong kind of bird. They strip-search you when you get here—not exactly squat and cough, but they do mean *naked*. It's weird having your belongings taken away and accounted for—a checklist from the life that brought you in here. It's weird not to know when you might leave.

We can actually see the outside world when we go to meals. I always want to sit closer to the window, but the others say it makes them sad. When we go to the playground, I'm back to elementary recess, the swings taking me so high, causing giggles to erupt from my mouth, my face dappled in sunshine. For the first time as an adult, I am reminded of a version of myself that is long gone. There's really no formula. From pregnant fourteen-year-olds to seventy-year-old homeless men, this is the common ground regardless of race, wealth, education, religion, or family makeup.

✧◆✧

There are people who say and do heinous things all over this planet, who really play at creating monstrous situations for those around them without a drop of pity or a passing thought. But we're the ones in here. If you ask us, the world makes a lot less sense and is a lot more ruthless outside of here.

✧◆✧

Most of us worried about how we would explain our situations to others once we got out. Ironically, it was employers and other unrelated folk who posed the most worry. Unconditional love and all that, I guess. Though not everyone was met with compassionate understanding by their friends and family. Anger, a natural but completely unhelpful response, often occurred.

To be so harsh with someone who is deeply depressed does as much good as rubbing a dog's face in poop after the deed has been done. Do you really think the dog doesn't know what shit smells like? That he didn't just create it and—bad dog!—shouldn't have gone right in the middle of the living room? We know what we did. We've just lost the ability to care. We can't help it.

One man who had turned himself in shared the secret of what he tells people on the outside. "I just say I had a bad reaction to some medication and had to go to the hospital for a while for them to sort it out."

It was perfect, and we filed it away for later use.

✧◆✧

This story starts with me handcuffed in the back of a sheriff's car while "Hotel California" blasts. It doesn't look good, I know. Picture it—a bright spring day, a gleaming cruiser, some chunky handcuffs joined to the chain around my waist, and "Hotel California" blaring through the car as we pulled away from one hospital to drive to another. We landed in a military town, and the Eagles kept crooning—over and over—in my head. The lyrics rang loud and true in my mind: I could check out whenever, but I could never leave.

DEPUTY JONES: She looked small and lost, but we've had to handcuff the elderly, children even. It's procedure. I try not to stop when transporting but knew I had to this time. "Do you need to use the restroom?" I ask.

"No, thank you," she replies.

I stare into the back seat a moment longer. She doesn't seem like a threat, but then again, you can't trust anyone in her position because they are so unpredictable.

"I still have to take you with me," I say.

I pull into a welcome center teeming with families of small children. It's May and the dogwoods are in full bloom. She looks about my age, and I think about how, under different circumstances, we could just be two friends out on a road trip.

I'm in the stall of the family restroom that has a bench when I hear the door push open. My charge is seated on the bench. I hear the clink of metal as she tells the woman that the stall is occupied. "C'mon, Timmy. Someone's in there," the woman says.

Based on the response, I envision a done-up lady, her voice an octave too high to be natural, with a small toddler at her side. Great, let's scar some families while we're at it.

We stand outside in the sunshine as I light my cigarette and try to make small talk. We discuss the weather and the number of tourists at this rest stop. We do not discuss the future. She shuffles a tiny bit away from me, and I get the impression she doesn't smoke. I don't know if I will see this particular one again, but I do know I'll shuffle back and forth from this place many more times this month. She doesn't seem like she could hurt people; these acts are done out of desperation just as much as violence.

✧◆✧

The Last Resort was a misnomer. It was neither the grand, bricked-in estates of decades past where terror hid behind the walls nor a technologically svelte resort, a more sterile hotel or home away from home. Instead, it was a placid building with a jumble of used and donated books in the cramped space of the so-called library and too much shellac over the wooden floors. It was an institution, no more, no less. Lex craned her neck, expecting to hear screams as she sat in the processing room with all the paperwork detailing health insurance, patient rights, and restrictive measures.

"You eat anything yet, honey?" the front desk clerk asked her.

"No," she said.

The clerk disappeared and returned ten minutes later with a foam box and cup, a spoon resting on top of the cup. The drink was red and smelled like sour water; the food was mostly unidentifiable—was that meat or cheese?—other than the green peas, easily scoopable for those without forks or knives. Lex looked pallid and anxious, like she wanted to claw her way back into the waiting room, into the real world. She was probably just tired, dazed, and hopeless though. Seafoam green attacked your eyeballs from all areas, and the chairs in the visitor's section had seen better days. They were the kind with printed fabric that had stains if you got up close and looked.

LEX: I cried the first night. And the second. I cried the third and fourth, and then the tears dried up. They'd come to me, well up, over the simplest thought. *What have you done? It's your fault you're in here. You have failed yet again. What will everyone think? How does this all end? You are unlovable.* The faces of all the people who didn't love me, weren't speaking to me, or had insulted me over the years came flooding back. I stared into the darkness and wept, too tired to think straight, too fearful to sleep. No one can save me this time.

My immediate thought, *I don't belong here,* rebuffed before the half-day's end. Maybe I didn't have multiple personalities or talk to myself or have mood swings so bad that no one could be around me, but the truth was plain. I needed to be there. I *did* belong there. Sure, I had my shit together—decent job, lots of education, homeowner—but all the signs of a normal life only highlighted how desperate I was. How unable I was to cope with pain on my own. How much I actually had to lose. There was no fight left in me, no denial. I knew why I was there. Even if most of the professionals I'd met didn't like to use the word "suicide."

The cruel trick of the social worker's betrayal was all that bothered me. She acted like the agreed-upon plan (my preferred plan) was to get me home instead of into an institution. But then she came back and said no, I couldn't go home. Was it because my therapist was out of the state? They had all the details up front. Why had they changed their minds?

The first night, the feeling of gnarled inferiority rooted itself in my chest. *I want—*

It doesn't matter what you want.

I was blocked immediately, and it was the first healthy thought I had in years. It was startling to find myself thinking healthy thoughts, to shut myself down using rational logic instead of feeding the beast. It didn't make me happier, but it was a start. Trained professionals and meds could do the heavy lifting—I'd already made my own attempts over the years. I went after the daily goals with vicious zeal.

Day 1: Get through a whole day without comparing myself to others.

Day 2: Don't talk about work.

Day 3: Combat any negative self-talk with a compliment a loved one had given me.

I made backup strategies for when I failed at these. Time was weird in such a place—some days dragged by, some went pretty smoothly. The schedule was our all. Idle minds were the devil's playground, right? Was that what happened? Had the devil somehow snuck up and snatched us at our most vulnerable? We weren't paying bills, working on projects, or dropping kids off at school, but we all worried about it, arranged for it to happen in our absence.

Someone figured out how to work the TV, but when we saw the news, we almost wished it wouldn't work again. We could watch the same four movies in a loop, over and over again—sometimes we did—or just go to bed early, which meant saying goodnight and lying in bed, pretending to sleep every fifteen minutes when they came to check on us. Wouldn't want them to think the lack of sleep was a med disruption—not the incessant noise, shaft of light from the hallway, mysterious roommate, or overwhelming sadness that crushed us from all corners. Not knowing what my roommate was in for definitely kept me awake. On more than one occasion, she would ask, "Can you hear me talking to myself?"

No, I never did.

"Are you sure?"

At some point, it occurred to me that maybe she was *hoping* I had heard her because that meant it wasn't all in her head.

The group became tight-knit with a scuffle only breaking out now and again, usually over some piece of nonsense. One of them wanted a vegetarian meal, and it looked better than the rest of the food, so then everyone wanted a vegetarian meal. So-and-so accidentally used such-and-such's towel, so now such-and-such was upset he didn't have one.

Some of the workers spoke to us like children. They were earnest but should have asked more questions about how we've tried to cope. They didn't really get into why we were there. That was up to us to share. Some of the counselors were empathetic, pensive, and detail-oriented. Some of them just thought worksheets and breathing exercises were miracle cures while we sat around and rolled our eyes at these unhelpful tactics. The guy I had been seeing prior to my little trip to The Last Resort had uttered something in response to a quip I made about "no winning."

"I don't think there's winning or losing. The only way you lose is by quitting the game," he said with a far-off stare exposing his own trauma.

Since he was one of the smartest people I had ever known, I listened and decided long after we stopped speaking to quit the game. Ironically, I had given my leftover pain meds to the same man after a procedure he had. Instead, I intentionally took sixteen ibuprofen—it was meant to be twenty-three, but people caught me in the act—and swigged vodka. If I'd had the pain meds, I might be dead. It didn't seem like anyone had much use for me, and I thought my absence would be minimal and perhaps even help resolve some ongoing issues for others.

Desperately sad but hell-bent on the impromptu plan, I dug up my will and wrote a short note—nothing brilliant but certainly honest. I wanted them to know that I was sorry. That I had tried. That I loved them all. I wanted it to be a peaceful message but for them to know how burdened I felt. I didn't know this would end in me eating chicken with a spoon, having my shoelaces confiscated—it's procedure—and discussing Jim Butcher novels with people who, in another life, would have been my friends. I spent a lot of time thinking about the recidivism rates, how people who landed there once probably would again. Why? Wasn't one trip to hell enough? Though, I had not been an "other-sider," so I had to give them credit.

To me, there were three groups. The first group had suicidal thoughts or other triggers and were preemptively committed. The second group was committed during an attempt. And the third group had knocked themselves out and only found out afterward they were not dead. The third group had brushed shoulders with the grim reaper; they were "the other-siders." In the first and second group, you had either reached out yourself ("voluntary commitment") or someone had reached out on your behalf or maybe you lost your shit quite publicly ("involuntary commitment").

You sometimes wonder, What's gonna happen here? All the staid and disgusting images from media portraying mental health flash through your mind. Squalor, straightjackets, and nurses with pillbox hats and mean glints in their eyes. My expectations were low—I didn't want to be beaten or sexually abused in any way. Luckily, I landed somewhere nestled next to a residential area. It was a clean facility with people who respected your privacy—or as much privacy as crazy people can be granted. I get that we're an unpredictable lot, but my existence—and near demise—proves that a person can be both desperately self-loathing and picky, a lethal combination. They needn't worry about shoelaces, razors, or drain cleaner—for me, it's either pills or nothing. Technically, guns are faster, but I don't touch the things and don't dare to leave such a mess behind. I was going to turn on *The Shawshank Redemption* and let the world burn out.

✧◆✧

I'd like to say that I flew down the road in a blind rage—people in stories like these are always flying into blind rages—but the truth this time was I felt my facial expression go completely slack and my resolve harden. When I got home, I was going to kill myself.

For such an impromptu moment, I was thorough, as I got out the ibuprofen and poured a full cup of vodka with a splash of ginger ale—for flavor, of all things. It was this careful planning that got me in trouble later—the fact that my suicide note and will were laid out neatly on the coffee table next to the couch where they would find my hopefully peaceful body. My mind had never been at peace, so perhaps my body would be. I was going to watch a movie and drift off to the land of overdose.

As I sat there, finally calm in my resolve, no longer fearing death but shaky in my emotions, I cried and talked out loud to a God I had spent the better part of a decade denying. Nothing works like a foxhole.

SANDY: The problem if you're in a relationship, or want to be, is that practically no one will do. Because if you find someone who has their head together, they often can't relate to you. But if you choose someone of your ilk—well, stories don't usually end like *Benny and Joon*, at least not that I've seen.

LEX: I keep a mental list of those who have been considered "crazy" over time:
- those who thought the earth was round
- those who thought the earth was flat

- those who believed in god(s)
- those who did not believe in god(s)
- Semmelweis

The last is the tragically true story of the doctor by the same name who advised professionals in the medical field to wash their hands in order to decrease the mortality rate among patients. Due to this fervent belief, he ended up dying in an insane asylum.

So that's how much we know.

✧◆✧

Most people are understandably upset to be in here, to be stripped of their creature comforts, civil liberties, and personal choices. And visitation—they're mad about their loved ones having to travel long distances to come see them for an hour, like we're in a zoo. Visitation is hard, but the rest of it—what to wear, when to eat—just gives me less to worry about. Whether or not I agree with their methods, I acknowledge that not having access to a computer or cell phone, for instance, must have some impact on helping us get out of here. That's the goal. When that door locks behind us, we're not checking into the Hilton. Some people call this acceptance wise—others just call it complacency.

#**58301:** I'd been at the big hospital for two days when Sandy got there. The big hospital is the first place they take you. You wait there, sometimes for days, until they find you a bed at a mental health facility they can transport you to while you wear handcuffs. At the big hospital, we're all roommates divided up by curtains unless or until you can get a private room. When Sandy got there, I caught her eye and said hello—just wanted somebody to talk to. Talking to people helps block out that voice in my head—okay, *urge*, like a normal kind of voice—that tells me to hurt myself. Usually, I find others to talk to, but they always go away. We exchanged what we were in for, and I was shocked she was not a student—too old even to be a traditional med student—and a survivor of an attempt. I hadn't done shit about my urge yet. I thought she was a sophomore like me.

Her eyes looked worried as she agreed to play War with me. I polished off the brownie on my tray. We played cards, and I told her I really just wanted her to talk to me. You couldn't just talk to anybody. You had to be able to talk to somebody who would converse with you, someone who was really there. She was nice enough but nervous. Right then, security came by and told me it was shower time. They escorted me out to a single stall shower where they gave me what little preapproved toiletries were allowed. By the time I got back, Sandy was back in her bed.

"Sandy," I whispered to her as I paused by her bed.

Nothing—she was already asleep. Maybe because in here you can't tell when it's night or day except for the clock on the wall. Even then, we wouldn't know if it was a.m. or p.m. if it weren't for the type of food that showed up on our trays. We're stuck in the basement of life, cut off from the outside world with no technology, like phones or computers, to tell us it was time to call grandma or alert us to the fourteen new texts our best friend sent. No celebrity gossip, weather forecasts, phone apps, or games—that part wasn't so bad actually.

Luckily, a new person arrived—straight out of detox/ rehab—and she was placed between Sandy and me. Her mascara was smudged heavily around her eyes, and she looked like she'd been through hell. Her dingy sweatpants and dingier blond hair somehow told me she had not come to this place willingly. Whew, that girl could talk!

"I just don't want to be left alone, you know?" she said.

"Girl, we're about to become best friends," I said. I just don't want to be left alone either.

SANDY: I wanted to be alone. I wasn't unfeeling or unfriendly toward those around me, but remembering where I was combined with the overwhelming need to get home was making me edgy. The kid, a decade younger than me, was smart, gifted really, but the fact that he seemed even more out of it than I was spoke to me and said, *Go to bed now.* There really wasn't much else to do anyway but lie there and wait out what was coming.

I sweated into the sheets, read the one awful book I could find, and waited. I didn't want to cause any trouble or be a bother, but I also wasn't here to make friends. I watched and listened as people screamed into the landline we all shared, spoke of gunshot wounds, and paced aimlessly. One young man approached the nurse's station to take his meds and locked eyes with an older guy who was standing across the hall. The older guy moved closer. "How you doing, Pop?" The pair hadn't seen each other in over a decade. No longer in the ER but not quite in my destination, I just wanted to be able to fall asleep and wake up to a world where I hadn't done the crazy things I did, where I didn't feel the way I always felt.

There are a lot of ways to kill yourself. No need to make a list—all the media we watch and people we encounter will fill that in for us. But for as long as I can remember, whenever I heard about someone offing themselves, my initial reaction, after sympathy, was, "That's not a good way to go." The pain, the mess, the agony. My way mostly ends poorly, too, when people have to get their stomachs pumped, and they are vomiting profusely.

Dark, the outside says. *Insane*. But, despite what the laws of nature, man, and God may say, I can't help but feel as though the right to end your life is just that—your right. Sure, it may affect the ones you love, cause a crisis in the medical field, and threaten your place in heaven, but, at the end of it all, most people who die by suicide aren't doing it to be selfish, thoughtless, dramatic, or vengeful. They're doing it because they can't see any way out of their predicament. That doesn't make them shortsighted because their predicament is not external— though that certainly drives it. Their predicament is that they hate themselves and don't know how to stop.

✧◆✧

I didn't think I belonged there—if I could cling to the workers, then I would be safe and wouldn't have to admit I was one of *them*. That strategy didn't last very long. Once, I fell asleep before group only to wake halfway through, peppering the conversation with my active participation. Everyone knew you had to participate to get out. Maybe because that was the only solid form of progress they could measure, scans for the soul and heart not being invented yet. We had yoga and badminton, but it was no country club. I peered in at the residential students—so young and malleable, already adrift. These kids, ages five to sixteen, mostly lived there year-round and received classroom learning during the day. I couldn't imagine teaching kids in such an environment and what particular challenges would crop up that would be more serious than note passing or copying of each other's homework.

✧◆✧

Everybody says they just want me to be happy, but what's the obsession with happiness? I can *feel* happy; I just can't *be* happy. Not in this lifetime. We all ask ourselves this from time to time: Am I capable of being happy? Am I capable of loving? Of being loved? Am I lovable? Some I immediately reject—my problem is that I can't stop loving. Some dog breeds have such a bite force that when their jaws clamp shut on what they are after, nothing can pry them apart short of breaking the dog's jaw. This is often the way love works with me.

When we hear criticism about ourselves, it's not a dispute in our head. It's more a sinking feeling of "Oh, you saw that too?" A feeling that others are homing in on exactly what you've hated about yourself all along. It's a strange illness; everyone feels so desperately alone, stranded in an abyss of hopelessness, and yet there we are all together. Perhaps misery really does love company—there's something more cathartic about group suffering at the hands of this cruel world. I felt tired while I was in there though. Dreadfully tired.

✧◆✧

People—the ones they call "normal"—may assume that someone who is ill is unreliable. They're not the Girl Scout troop leader, the pastor, or the CEO of a Fortune 500 company. They're going to assume that the highly responsible and smiling are even-keeled.

✧◆✧

Get up, get dressed, take meds. Go to work, work, don't work. Come home, read, take meds, go to bed. Rinse and repeat with variation here and there: go to the gym, pet the cats, see a movie. But it all starts the same: get up, get dressed, take meds. Without that, there is no beginning. At least my showers are longer than thirty seconds now. Developing a sense of self-worth is more challenging than people perceive it to be. They think it's a matter of pulling from an internal well, but this well was filled with external water—a conveniently forgotten aspect.

It isn't until much later that I realize I've walked out on my life in many ways. Three jobs, two schools, and one relationship. Over and over again, I am the quitter I never sought to become. Between the unwieldy desire to be elsewhere and my proactive rejection to spare my own feelings, I've somehow become a Dharma Bum. Me—

once filled with so much drive I didn't know the meaning of rest. Anything is possible, I guess. Now I only know the meaning of restlessness.

DEPUTY JAMES: I remembered her face right away.

LEX: There's no way she remembered me. They've seen hundreds of people since then.

DEPUTY JAMES: Of course, we're not allowed to say anything unless we're approached first. Still, seeing people who went through that at all must be a positive sign, right? Better than the alternative. It's a perk of the job, for sure.

LEX: She has no idea how much her kindness helped make that miserable moment better for me. How I never wanted cops on duty in my place, and suddenly I brought them right to my door, tramping through my living room and dining room. How far those few, kind words went to, if not normalize the situation, at least begin my intense journey with some empathy.

DEPUTY JAMES: I wonder if she still lives in the same place—section A, division D on our maps—if she's doing any better. My sister always puts me on call when one of those cases comes up, says I'm good at it, that it runs in the family. "If that's so true, why can't you go?" I'd ask. She just shakes her head, her lips halfway between a smile and a grimace. So, I go.

H.D.: I tell them to picture a peaceful scene. It sounds hokey, and usually when people hear me say that, they make a face and try to conjure up images of soft waves lapping the sand or deep meditation in a near-silent wood. This is not what this exercise is for. Though, in all truth, I'll take any image that settles them down and calms their frayed nerves—whatever's most helpful to them. But secretly, the practitioner in me hopes they'll think of a challenging situation and how they would confront it to make their own peace. Not a revenge fantasy—that's never the goal, though they can be outrageously funny—but some healthy, realistic way to manage their broken lives.

"Picture a peaceful scene in your mind."

#66921: Just one day where they don't call me trash.

#80912: A good, long smoke.

LEX: This question makes me nervous …

#63630: Walking around in sweats, a drink in my hand. Just a quiet night.

#28439: She calls and says she loves me.

#58301: New friends, ones that don't try to get me to use.

LEX: What does peace look like?

✧◆✧

Some of my friends really cracked me up. A couple of girls would stand on the sidelines with me during rec, and we'd observe each person. A throwback to recess and tag and crushes, before we knew better. One guy stood across the courtyard by himself, taking it all in. His eyes were shockingly blue and his hair perpetually tussled. Looking at him was like inhaling smoke and seeing mirrors.

LEX: He's cute.

#63630: Really cute.

LEX: Right. He's probably crazy.

#63630: Not everyone's crazy.

LEX: That seems like a large statement.
(Silence)

LEX: His eyes look like they've seen things.

#63630: Well, I can think of a few more things I'd like him to see.
(Laughter)

✧◆✧

In real life, I wear makeup and dresses and high heels. Here, during art therapy, they have us make collages from ratty, unfashionable magazines sporting businesses that went out of style about twenty years ago. We have to rip since scissors aren't allowed.

"Eww," one guy says.

"What?" I ask. He is sniffing a perfume ad. I pull it from his hands and laugh. "That's what I wear in the real world!"

Outside, I have always had a very firm idea of what my life should be. I was ambitious and sober. I thought I could rearrange the laws of physics that make a rubber band snap. There were so many days of wasted potential. So many days of wondering what the hell the point was. It was bound to happen sooner or later—at least, that's the way I feel about it.

✧◆✧

I'm going to have my loved ones drive three hours just to see ... what? That I'm still here? No, thank you. The harpoon of guilt already twists itself in my gut enough without adding yet another interruption to their lives. Sixty minutes of pitying eye contact and cooing words is not my idea of love while I'm in here. I'm fascinated watching those I know speak with their visitors, but somehow, I feel cagey and defensive about my incarceration. Besides, there's always the once-a-day phone call, and that's one I'll never miss.

✧◆✧

They give us worksheets to fill out with questions on them. Do you tend to:
- stuff your anger? *Not really*
- avoid direct confrontation? *No*

- tell yourself it's unreasonable to be optimistic? *Yes*
- try to control yourself but escalate to rage? *Yes*

They teach us about emotional insulation and intellectualization. They teach us the danger of rhetorical questions in the mouths of others and how we can only be responsible for our own actions. At the end, there's a chart with sixteen negative responses to stress—I circle twelve of them. Nobody wants to cheat off me. I've got all the wrong answers.

I don't think it's normal, but sometimes I understand why some people want nothing to do with other humans.

#19145: Some of us have secrets so dark we don't even want to admit them to ourselves. Apparently, this is called "repression" ... or "regression." Same thing.

SANDY: If someone told you your skin was blue, would you believe them? What if they told you sixty times? Six hundred times? What if several people started to tell you that? All the people you care about? Would you believe them?

LEX: The toothbrush was made of some kind of corn product like the eco-utensils at my college. The kind of plastic that doesn't even break when you bend it. Every morning, I tried brushing my teeth without ending up with a half-bent toothbrush, like I had Superman's strength.

SANDY: That's what people felt like to me, a hydra of disapproval. Maybe it's because you wear your hair short or the reason you wear your hair short. Maybe it's because you're overweight or the reason you're overweight. Maybe it's because you have night terrors or the reason you have night terrors. You can be as smart, good-looking, kind, and funny as you want. You can be anything you want, they say. They lied, though, because I can't be yours.

LEX: I took account of my surroundings. In hospitals, the idea is to duplicate the home experience, almost like a hotel. That's why waiting areas all look like hotel lobbies or living rooms—artwork on the wall, patterned carpeting, soft lighting, and the inevitable box of tissue placed just so. Aesthetics didn't factor in much at the institution.

I understood the casual, understated attitude toward me when I saw certain cases. People were literally trying to escape by stealing the badges off hospital workers, and then you just had sorry sack me who wanted an extra bottle of water. "You could have really done damage to your kidneys or other organs had you taken the amount of ibuprofen you did for several days in a row," the admitting doc warned. Could he hear himself? He was preaching quality of life to someone who wanted to end it all in one evening. Not a bad guy but certainly not the sharpest.

At the physical hospital, one I had never been to, they let me run around without socks and neglected to take off my wire leads, which were long enough to drape over the hook of the bathroom door to choke myself— if I were so inclined. And this was one of the better hospitals—it wasn't bad, just inconsistent. How the general population expects crazy people—reclaiming the pejorative—to function in an unstable world is beyond me. One passing patient developed lumps on his head and arms for no reason. "Worry lumps" he called them. He beat them out of himself every chance he got. For some reason, it's the ones with dark hair and light eyes that are most unmanageable.

✧◆✧

We shared our daydreams of what we would do once we left. Drinking, eating our favorite foods, wearing makeup, having sex, and shaving led the pack of fantasies we told ourselves.

#19145: Something dislodges in your chest, and your mind begins to unspool.

I am incredibly well-adjusted! Followed by laughter because it's true.

Yet as a culture, we eat seaweed and charcoal and chlorophyll and grasshoppers. We plank and take pole-dancing classes, do hoopilates, engage in a fitness program ironically called Insanity. We pay money to trap ourselves in a humid room—the likes of Florida in the dead of summer—to bend ourselves like pretzels and chant words we don't know the history of. We turn to cloning and cryogenic freezing, to shamans and deities. So many people running around trying to avoid death at any cost. People who never learned the meaning behind "If you can't beat 'em, join 'em." We're just a subset, I suppose.

✧◆✧

Trauma: When someone else's heart turns to ice, but it's your blood that runs cold.

SANDY: People have interesting reactions to learning you've been in the loony bin. Some act like they didn't hear you and just keep texting about the mundane details of their day, an aversion to serious topics of conversation and certainly a barrier to growing intimacy with someone. Others try to normalize it, never cracking their unruffled veneer, to the extent that they must realize their unnatural, unflappable reaction makes them seem weirder than the person confessing. Most people offer pithy apologies and platitudes of thankfulness that you're fine—then they go back to the mundane details route.

It's obviously an uncomfortable topic for most, just like anything associated with death—unless it's fictional, because we love to watch people getting killed in TV shows and movies—a distancing of oneself from the inevitable. We crazies burn bright like a fire. Others skirt our edges, so they won't get burned, as though depression were contagious like the flu or herpes.

"What led you to want to end your life?"

"How did it happen?"

"Do you want to talk about it?"

All are acceptable and understandable questions, yet seldom are these details sought, which in turn, does not provide the former patient, now everyday citizen of the world again, with the opportunity to talk about it, their experience, their woes. As Dinah Shore said, "Trouble is part of your life—if you don't share it, you don't give the person who loves you a chance to love you enough." Turns out, it depends on who you're sharing it with.

My friend had a therapist once who, after addressing my friend's concerns that their diagnosis was incorrect, promptly evaluated and diagnosed her a second time and then rushed to add, "I'm sure that's true, but I'm not going to focus on it." A complete acknowledgment and dismissal in one breath. The therapist probably thought that by putting the patient first rather than the diagnosis, they were respecting the whole person and preventing the patient—my friend—from getting stuck on labels rather than treatment. But what if my friend *wanted* to talk about this shift in diagnosis? She had waited a long time—over a decade—to find out what was wrong with her and felt some relief in hearing it was something established.

#19145: It's hard to outrun the past when you're still creating it.

Like a kid who sets their heart on one day becoming a veterinarian, some people never wanted to be anything but sane. With the fierce tenacity of a child wishing for a puppy, they put sanity on their Christmas list each and every year. Sanity is not a puppy, but the hope is that it can be housebroken, groomed, and trained accordingly. That it can be taken out for a stroll around the neighborhood whenever necessary.

LEX: Each person is served court papers the day you're processed through. Basically, after your first week there, you must sit before a lawyer so they can assess your situation and condition and give the stamp of approval on your retainment or release.

"I thought I didn't have to go?"

"There might have been a delay in paperwork. It's fine. It won't affect when you get to go home."

I reluctantly followed the aid back to a small, hidden room where a rather grouchy lady sat before me. She had gray dreads and spoke in a gruff, clipped way, even though she was using terms like "darling." She meant me no harm.

"I see you came in wanting to hurt yourself," she stated. She made notes the whole time she spoke, barely looking up into my face every now and again. I wondered if this was pro bono work for her. "Is that still the case?"

"N-no," I stammered. "I feel much better. The stay's been helpful," I added. Her eyes, bullshit detectors, could tell I was not lying.

"Oh," she interrupted our interview. "I see you're due to leave today," she added with some surprise. "You're good to go. Take care of yourself."

✧◆✧

What percentage did the mass amount of people who weren't allowed to vote account for? Did sons and daughters who had birthdays while their parents were inside stay the same age, frozen in time? Would they cancel Mother's Day too? Would your job hold your position for a month? Your college your homework for a year? We tried to turn the news on once, but it was too depressing.

✧◆✧

When I visit the art museum, I see large bodies looming in bronze and marble, fine rudimentary figures crafted from teakwood, and oil smeared on canvas depicting both the royalty and peasants of the time. So much emphasis on the body, the corporeal, as though one could not disentangle the spirit from the shell, the container, the ever-eroding, malfunctioning, sometimes useful and fun packaging that comes without lifetime guarantee and a very strict expiration date. It's easy to see how the two get confused, curled up in each other like a Russian nesting doll, indecipherable between the cargo and the ship itself. The hopes for college admittance are thought by the young brain, the fear of a wild animal approaching felt by a quickened pulse. The gaze of love disturbing our loins and the Pavlovian response to hunger. Once a rumble in the belly is now a pleasant feeling of anticipation and satisfaction. Our emotions, thoughts, and soul—our very being, our personality—are housed within the body and cannot escape. To release one is to release the other …

#19145: The lisp of the heart, the incorrect pronunciation of a love gone wrong.

✧◆✧

Great lines of cars moving up and over the hills like giant centipedes.

✧◆✧

You lack the self-esteem, self-discipline, self-confidence, sense of self that you not only richly deserve but need to get by in this brutal place we call Earth. You have a slew of other problems—you're only fun when you're high, you're only high when you're fun. Your only purpose or meaning is tied to money, love, another person, your physique. You've been told a thousand times, directly and indirectly, this is your only worth.

There are barrages of functioning compulsive liars out there. We even lie to ourselves. I know I do.

LEX: We are chained, one foot shackled to the other, the mind balancing back and forth between the two, our personality and thoughts distorted and warped before one day, something breaks and cannot be glued back together. There may be those who die from spite, jealousy, revenge, self-appointed martyrdom, a sense of control over others, but I've not met them. You think you can get by and fix yourself because that is what we're taught at every turn, but just like rescuing a beached whale or dancing the waltz, some things were not meant to be done alone.

✧◆✧

Love kills. So does grief, loneliness, and lack of hope. Pride, joining love, is another one of those supposedly positive experiences that falls apart, the inverse being failure, the inverse of love being rejection or loss.

✧✦✧

Just in the way we wish to sweat out fat, if I could sweat out the nightmares, the anxiety, the constant self-doubt, I would. I'd pour myself into lemonade pitchers too small to fit my essence.

✧✦✧

When I got out, I heard "Hotel California" everywhere—buskers at the mall, department stores, and always in the car. It was true. This was an experience that I could never leave. There were a few key friends I needed to come clean with once I got home. We tried to have a dinner, but only half of them could make it—further proof that the world spins on without you. I used my best material, tried to tell them about the ridiculous chicken/spoon episode, but it only made them cry harder. They were relieved to see me but dismayed and worried that I had gotten to that point at all. Sooner or later, something in life breaks you—an accident, an infidelity, a tragic and abrupt halt to the person you once were even if the newer version is wiser, if not worse for the wear. We all have our breaking points, and I had far exceeded mine.

✧✦✧

I was out with my boyfriend at the time, shopping for a card. I can't even remember the occasion now.

"Our thoughts are with you …"

"You're the BEST uncle in the world!"

"I've loved you since the moment I saw you …"

I just remember feeling surrounded, smothered under the array of memories and emotions the cards provoked in me.

"CONGRATULATIONS! You did it!"

"There are no words to express how sorry I am ...

... a birthday you'll never forget."

Barely able to breathe, I closed my eyes.

"Hey ... hey, are you all right, baby?"

"No," I sobbed adamantly. I didn't care that I was crying in the middle of the aisle or who saw me. My anger and pain bundled together, at once inseparable. "I'm not okay! Why would you ask that?"

"You can talk to me. You were fine a minute ago. Nothing's happened since then, right?"

I wiped at a snot bubble. His concern felt surface level. "You don't understand!" I blurted. A lady with salt-and-pepper hair looked our way.

"Let's go home and talk about it," he whispered.

"Why? Because you're so worried about what other people think? You want me to hide how I'm feeling! They matter more?" I retorted loudly. That old familiar emptiness curled itself inside my chest and smashed me over and over and over again. The few shreds of identity I'd found over the last ten years were just that— smithereens, pieces of disparate puzzles that would never meld together. Standing there, among all those cards, I felt the utter hopelessness of my condition, of my insignificant life. When we pulled up at home, I let myself inside then locked myself in the bedroom and didn't come out for the next two days.

❖◆❖

There were so many things. The ongoing fights with my cousin, being dumped mercilessly—a shotgun to a dog's head—by the only man I'd fallen in love with during the last decade, the lack of progress in my spiritual, professional, financial, vocational life. My best friend moving across the country. I couldn't point to one thing really.

❖◆❖

We buzzed like a swarm of bees at phone-call time every night. We weren't supposed to loiter around the nurse's station, but we did anyway. Calls were limited to five minutes, but sometimes, when things were slow and no one was making a ruckus, they allowed each of us a little extra time on the phone, upward of ten minutes. There was nowhere private to take the cordless phone and not more than one chair in the hallway, so people loped up and down or crouched in a corner to exact some amount of privacy instead. Most calls were short and sweet, maybe a catch-up of what was happening on the outside, an updated status of what the person on the other end was doing to free the person counting off their days inside the psych hospital. A few people came back visibly rattled, red-faced and puffy from spilled tears. We always held our breath to see who would pick up, and sometimes nobody was home. You could try again or try a different number, but if you were too much out of luck, then you'd have to wait one more day. I called my brother, the one person other than my boyfriend who I trusted to not judge me for being involuntarily committed to such a place. At the end of his calls, my brother told me he loved me, and I felt verklempt, knowing that it wasn't something he said lightly.

✧◆✧

I'm told it's harder the older you get because you have less and less time to make things right.

✧◆✧

There are large coloring pages we can use that have optimistic slogans plastered all over them, a board game or two, and a stack of magazines with old hair and makeup tips.

✧◆✧

Donella is old. She could be in her sixties or seventies. But if I saw her on the street, I would place her at eighty or ninety. She has a soft, whispery voice and a shriveled frame, but she does not seem scared of much. She's fragile but in an assertive way.

"I can't wait to get back and make some of my glory brownies. I make them with Carliff, my grandson. He just *loves* him some glory brownies! Have I told you about these brownies before?"

"No, I don't think so," I respond with a small smile. She has mentioned them at least twice but has never gone into any detail of what makes them earn the title of glorious.

"Well, you bake them with crushed hazelnuts inside, and you slice them real thin …"

My mouth has already started to water, and I can smell hazelnuts in the air as I envision the perfectly moist brownie with a flaky, crusty layer. She has stopped talking. Donella turns to me.

"Do you think they'll let me bake again?"

I see the sadness in her eyes. I rub her upper back softly. "Of course," I say in what I hope is a comforting tone. They ask if there are any guns in our homes but don't think of the knives we use to cook, pills for migraines, belts to complete outfits, or drain cleaner to unclog our pipes. Anything can be a weapon when you're desperate enough. "I don't know the exact rules, but of course they'll let you bake again. They can't regulate us on the outside." And I know what I've spoken is both a blessing and a curse.

✧♦✧

Night-rounds-guy has a limp we all notice but don't mention until later when we see him wearing shorts. That's when we discover he has a prosthetic lower leg. We look upon him as a positive sign that the facility employs those who are "different," and it makes me wonder about phantom limbs. Isn't that just a trick of the mind? If so, how different is that from any of the other tricks our minds play on us? Why is one so widely acknowledged while the others are ostracized or exoticized? My mind outpaces itself. That's the problem with me—I never know when to stop.

✧◆✧

My mom used to say, "Don't talk to yourself, you look crazy." Now am I qualified to? At this time—I have nothing *but* time in The Last Resort—I could talk to myself out loud all I want, but I've never done so less. The mutterings of to-do items and breathy curses are suddenly gone from my daily existence.

✧◆✧

I suggest we watch a movie, only to realize too late the therapist is the villain. Oops.

✧◆✧

Everyone's got a pithy remedy when you're sick in the head. The difference between recommending chicken soup for a cold and endlessly licking your wounds is people saying, "If you'd only exercise, focus on the positive, keep a gratitude journal, go to church, eat better, sleep more, drink more water, work less, work harder, do community service, get involved, join a club, make a change, move, quit your job, break up, get an online dating profile, visit your family more, cut negative people out, cut carbs out, cut sugar out, make a vision board, take a class …"

As though we could will ourselves back into health, into happiness. As though, if we just strive hard enough, then our whole life will come together and nothing bad can touch us. We'll feel okay about anything and instantly know how to cope. We'll see the grand design of it all, the painful utility behind the plan, why everything happens for a reason. Crying is unnatural. Screaming is unnatural. Meds are unnatural. Sleeping twelve plus hours a day—out of the question. The problem is, while we're running around tending each part of our lives, something is slipping further and further out of view, and a different piece breaks. So we rush to fix that and in doing so, neglect ourselves and our emotions once again. It's an endless setup for failure.

Clara, a neighbor who lived at the end of our cul-de-sac, did all these things. Her life was run like a Rockwellian vision of Americana, all the way down to the white picket fence. She had a career she loved and was both a PTA mom and church leader. Clara went to the gym three times a week and routinely got mistaken for being a decade younger than she was. Even her blood pressure, height, and shoe size were average. She balanced her work responsibly, and day after day she toiled for five years before receiving a promotion. She came home one day to her family, unlocking the door in the garage, then remembered she left her lunch box out in the car. She returned to the car, unlocked it, sat inside, started the engine, shut the garage door, and proceeded to fume herself out of this world. Her obituary read, in part, that "Clara Honore was a steady, dependable person."

✧◆✧

I could have been more faithful,
more strung out on belief.
I could have made smarter decisions.
I could have been more disciplined,
been more practical.

I could have stayed, could have left,
could have given up,
or could have stuck with it.
This is the prayer of the lost.

#19145: All the Southern men I know say "bye" in the same way. A clipped syllable. A soft, open-ended purr. It never sounds final.

✧◆✧

My friends hide, sequestered from the truth. I like to take it out into the light and beat it until it cries uncle.

✧◆✧

"A method to the madness," they say. I have news for them though. If there's a method, then it's not madness. You can call it whatever you'd like—institution, sanitorium, mental hospital, psychiatric facility, nuthouse, funny farm, loony bin, insane asylum, madhouse, booby hatch, snake pit, psycho ward, bedlam. It's still good old-fashioned madness at the end of the day.

LEX: Music was big for us in Cellblock Four West. We brought a radio or begged for a worker to plug their phone into a speaker everywhere we went. There would be dancing at times, but mostly we just liked the reminder of something pleasant from the outside world. We were waiting in the cafeteria line one day when Everclear came on the radio. "Oh shit," I said.

"What?" my friend asked.

"If I weren't here right now, I'd be seeing them tonight. I'm supposed to be in Oregon on vacation, and we had concert tickets ... shit," I responded. The irony washed over me as the lunch lady sloshed gravy onto my mashed potatoes.

✧◆✧

When coming back in from the courtyard, sometimes I would try to open the door only to be reminded that it was locked to me, that I was at the mercy of someone else. This filled me with incongruent rage. That something as simple as a *door* should be a barrier to me was inconceivable. This effect would last, even in my outside life, and I would blink slowly while inhaling, tamping down the anger.

✧◆✧

The hospital wasn't a Shangri-La of acceptance, heralding in my days as a more carefree individual. When I left, I was still fractured but much less so. I was considering myself and my life in a much different light, possibly for the first time in my adulthood. I was forced to sit with myself and realize maybe I wasn't the hopeless monster I feared I'd become. Doing so sharply brought to my attention the silliest of joys throughout the day.

I heard squeaky voices saying nonsense words as a few of my friends gathered around one of the counselors. My feet followed, and soon I was watching some stupid sock puppet videos online and giggling like they were the funniest things in the world. It didn't even make sense. The videos were little more than color and noise, but that's what made them so ridiculous. All these pointless human creations I had forgotten about or ignored—maybe there was a little sunshine after all.

We formed the sheer habit of getting to know one another through the countless hours we had to share our preferences, our histories, our triggers, and the pieces of ourselves we were so apt to hide away from others on a regular basis. These were connections I could not ignore—should not ignore. Relating to others on a real level when so much of what we do is polite or fake is a gift without a receipt. These people were seeing me at my absolute worst and still accepting me. They were focusing in on what matters, not the trappings but the personality. Even then, it was hard to believe I deserved as much. I had disappointed everyone and when push came to shove, didn't really believe in myself, so I deserved whatever I got. That was the thinking I was trapped in before.

It wasn't all funny videos and conversation that cheered me though. Learning and knowing that my circumstances may not change but that *I* had changed and could change was huge. Just by my attempt alone, I had taken myself seriously and committed to something. Maybe others who knew would take me seriously too. Even though a large part of my goal-oriented nature seemed to fall to the side, it hadn't; my goals had just changed. One of the thoughts that constantly stuck with me and made me feel more positive was that there was a way out and, therefore, a goal. *You will get out of this hospital, and you will not come back*. My spirits were buoyed—being myself out in the real world and trying my best were just going to have to be enough.

SANDY: I paced up and down the hallways. Three laps, four laps, five. That clock would just not speed up at all. My boyfriend was late for everything, and this just about proved it, but I didn't care. I knew this would be my last day at The Last Resort. I knew it wasn't raining, knew it was probably one thousand degrees outside, and I wanted to feel the sun crackle on my skin, burn it and turn it to deep shades of pink. I wanted out from the bad fluorescent lighting, constant ease of temperature, and bland-colored walls—beyond. I wanted beyond. I beyond wanted. When Dorothy Gale arrives in Munchkinland and the camera follows her path in brilliant Technicolor—this is how it felt. I was grateful but repulsed enough to never want to come back unless it was in a working capacity. I had escaped after a seven-day trick. I had faced down my inner demon, and instead of vanquishing it, I had come out being friends with it, understanding it more fully. When you are trying to be your best self, it helps to have your worst self around as a reminder. I knew one thing—they called me Lex, but Lex was gone.

#19145: The truth is a muddied thing. To begin with, there's so little of it.

ACKNOWLEDGMENTS

My sincerest thanks to Mindy Kuhn, Amy Ashby, Melissa Long, and the hardworking staff of Warren Publishing for their dedication. Special mention should go to the Honeysuckle Tea House and Wildwoods Community Farm in Chapel Hill, North Carolina. Unlike the rest of my work, most of this was written outdoors, so if it is found to be lacking, I blame the fresh air. Lastly, thank you to all the individuals who make up the mental health community and who strive day in and day out to help provide a better life for those with mental illness. If you ever wonder if you have made an impact, the answer is a resounding "yes."